Detox: How to Perform a General Cleaning of the Body

Everything You Need to Know about a Detox Diet and Metabolism

By Sandra Crosby

Table of Contents

Introduction

The dream of many people is to eat anything they want and not get fat.

Most people tend to be physically attractive and are also healthy.

However, not everyone manages to have both, even with great effort.

Do you limit yourself in everything, but can't seem to lose weight?

Not all modern food can be called healthy and safe. Many foods contribute to the deterioration of the body.

At the same time, when a person cannot lose weight even though they diet and limit the intake of high-calorie foods, it's because their metabolism is functioning poorly.

These two situations - the consumption of junk food and metabolic disorders - are interrelated; the second is a consequence of the first.

To lose weight with a slow metabolism, you need to restore its speed, and this will help the appropriate diet.

The results depend on the individual's initial physical figure and the neglect of metabolic problems.

Every person suffering from being overweight dreams of "painless" weight loss. Many are frightened by the very scary word "diet", which implies restriction and starvation. But people are weak in their whims. Particularly comforting is the idea that if you cannot eat it, but really want to, then you can eat just a little bit. And then a little more and again... So slowly but surely, we are gaining extra pounds, not knowing where they come from.

How do you get rid of excess weight, look great and feel energetic and strong?

Many modern diets help with this. Their purpose is to accelerate one's metabolic process. One such diet is the currently popular detox diet.

It may seem unusual, but this diet is not only aimed at losing weight.

Everyone has already heard about the harm of mono-diet, long-term unbalanced starvation diets and similar methods that help to lose weight, but at the same time undermine our health. The detox diet is primarily aimed at getting rid of toxins, and therefore results in the improvement of the whole body. Losing those extra pounds is only a nice bonus.

However, like any other diet, it has its pros and cons, which we will sort out this book.

Chapter 1: What Is Metabolism and Why Is It Important

Metabolism – Why Would Life without It Be Impossible?

A set of all vital processes that take place in our body is called metabolism. Simply put, these are all processes that influence the generation of energy required for the proper functioning of our organism. And to do this, we need to provide the body with enough "fuels," that is, quality nutrients. Our digestive tract is in charge of transforming foods we consume into the energy we need.

Starting from the basic actions, such as breathing and digestion of food, to more demanding processes such as the transmission of nerve impulses, our body needs the energy to perform all these actions. After we eat food, various digestive enzymes break down macronutrients into a form that our body can use over and over. So, long-term starvation is not an option, because the inflow of "fuel" must be permanent.

The quality of energy will depend on the food we consume. Proper and balanced selection of ingredients means that all useful nutrients can be extracted from them. That way, waste will be minimal. These are all toxic materials that can't become energy, and which are stored somewhere in our body.

Catabolism and Anabolism

All metabolic processes are divided into two groups - catabolism and anabolism.

Catabolism represents the decomposition of nutrients. This metabolic process involves a series of chemical reactions that break down complex compounds into smaller units. For example, complex carbs break into simple carbs, and proteins disintegrate into amino acids. During these processes, our body generates the energy it needs for growth, development, and sustenance.

Catabolism gives energy to our body, which is essential for not only performing all vital functions but also for doing physical activity. It is required, from the cellular level to the entire body movements. The energy that occurs in these processes is stored and represents fuel for anabolic actions.

While catabolism decomposes substances, anabolism creates them. That is precisely why the second name for this process is biosynthesis. Simple molecules are synthesized into more complex compounds and thus build muscles, tissues, bone mass, etc. Catabolism creates the energy anabolism consumes for the production of hormones, enzymes, sugars, and other cell growth agents.

If catabolism produces more energy than anabolism requires, there will be a surplus of energy. The human body stores this excess energy in the form of fat cells or glycogen. Unlike muscle tissues, which are the most active energy consumers, these fatty layers are inactive. They need energy just for maintenance of the existing form. More simply, it's unnecessary fat. In order not to create it, we need a balanced input of food that is abundant with nutrients, and which ensures optimal energy level.

When Metabolism Loses Its Function

A well-known medical myth is that skinny people have a faster metabolism than people with excessive weight. Reality is much different. Numerous studies have shown that slower metabolism, in most cases, is not the reason for someone's obesity. Metabolism depends on many factors, which you might not even have imagined.

We can't influence some of these factors, such as aging and gender. The older we are, we lose more muscle mass and increase the amount of fat. Less muscle means less energy consumption, and the metabolism slows down naturally. As for gender factor, men usually have a faster metabolism, because they are naturally bigger than women and have less fat.

And what is very important, is the genetic factor—some people just have the advantage that their metabolism is faster, while others, unfortunately, aren't that lucky.
However, we can influence other key factors like healthy nutrition, quality sleep, and regular physical activity. We should adapt food intake to our daily physical activity routine, and find a balance that will maintain the function of our organism at the optimal level.

Slow metabolism caused by one of these factors can lead to many health problems. Constant fatigue, the need for free sugar and empty calories (foods with no or very little nutrients), and often mood swings are just some of the clear signs that something is wrong with your metabolism.

Chapter 2: Health Conditions Caused by Disrupted Metabolic Function

Disturbance of metabolic function lead to many diseases, but it can also be the result of some changes in the body. Irregular elimination of toxins can endanger the flow of energy and slow down metabolism. When our body can't discharge toxins correctly, then we have to react.

Overweight

Blaming slow metabolism for the inability to lose weight can sound like an excuse for laziness and a weak character. But this claim is the truth. The factors that we can't control are partly responsible for slow metabolism. Some people have higher chances for this condition, and it prevents them from effective shedding of extra pounds.

However, proper functioning of metabolism is mainly the result of life habits. Although we can't prevent some of the effects, we can make them less reflective on our health. When our metabolism slows down, fat deposits grow faster. It may result in the appearance of a few extra pounds. If we change nothing in our eating or exercising routine, those few pounds can easily become chronic obesity. Further, it can cause more problems with the heart, liver, fertility, etc.

Constipation

Poor digestion is a common problem that can slow down metabolism. The difficulty of regular bowel discharge is the most frequent consequence of slow metabolism. If this condition is acute, it can be solved with various diets and probiotics. Over time, our body stores too much waste that can interrupt the discharge of the bowel. Therefore, as a means of prevention, it is desirable to apply detox diets from time to time.

Slowing metabolism leads to the appearance of sluggish bowel symptom, a condition where the digestive system just can't process food. If the condition becomes chronic, it is required to change nutrition and life habits. It can have significant consequences if we don't treat it in time. A well-timed visit to a doctor and nutritionists is a must when you notice this problem.

Chronic Fatigue

Chronic fatigue represents extreme exhaustion of the organism. This issue is the result of modern lifestyle, poor nutrition, and everyday stress. All mentioned factors are the causes of this condition, which requires urgent treatment because the sick person is not able to work, live or function normally.

Slow metabolism and toxins accumulated in the body affect our health in many ways. Poor digestion and irregular discharge of the bowel can cause the organism to weaken. All these waste materials stress and poison our body, and if something doesn't change, it won't function as before. People who suffer from chronic fatigue always feel exhausted and lifeless. This condition often leads to the appearance of some mental illnesses, as it significantly changes the life of the diseased person.

Chapter 3: How to Boost Your Metabolism Naturally

Although our metabolism slows down over the years, we can prevent its earlier occurrence with proper nutrition, sleeping, exercising and avoiding stressful situations. The normal metabolic function is not required just because of easier weight loss, but also because of the overall health condition.

By raising the quality of life and changing bad habits, we can reduce the risk of many diseases that can damage our health.

Many pharmaceutical agents can help us speed up metabolism, but there's no need for them. The use of drugs and preparations that promise magical results is often a waste of time and money. Not to mention the potential health risks. The treatment for metabolism boosting can be found in nature, even in our kitchen; it takes only a little knowledge and determination to bring some positive changes to our life.

Quality and Quantity of Food

The choice and quantity of foods affect not only the speed of metabolism, but also the rhythm and way of eating specific ingredients. For each group of nutrients, there is a precisely determined period of time when it should be eaten. Our digestive tract is a complex system, which includes many organs and enzymes required for the decomposition of food. It is logical that the organism will more easily digest raw or minimally processed food, rather than industrial products.

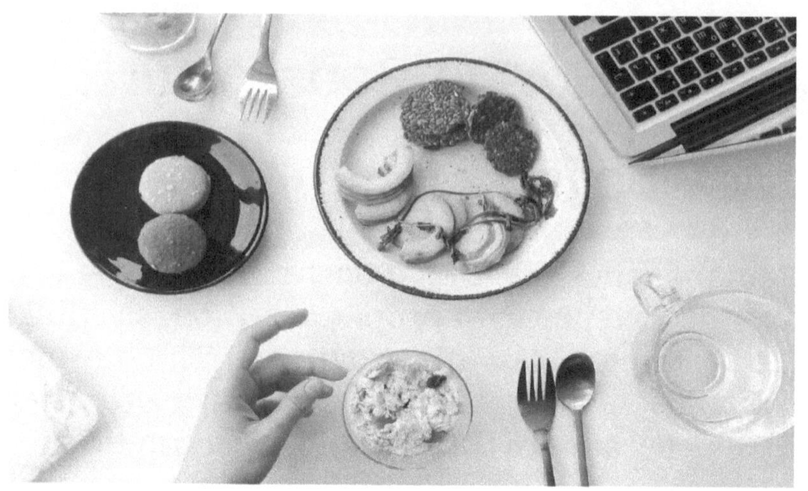

You may have noticed that if you eat right before bedtime, you have problems with the stomach, which also affects the quality of sleep. In the morning, you're usually tired and nervous, even if you've slept enough. As the day passes, the activity of our organs decreases; the digestive tract slows down in the evening, and digestion of heavy foods in this period, such as complex carbohydrates or saturated fats, will burden it. And even before the process of digestion is completed, you probably would have fallen asleep with a half-full stomach.

Starving Is Not an Option

Our body is active 24/7. For making that possible, the energy flow must be constant. Even when we do nothing, we need energy for basic physiological processes—it's called basal metabolism. The amount of energy our body consumes in the state of rest during the day is expressed by the BMR number and is the number of calories which basal metabolism burn. This is influenced by many factors, such as age, gender, the percentage of muscle mass, and health status.

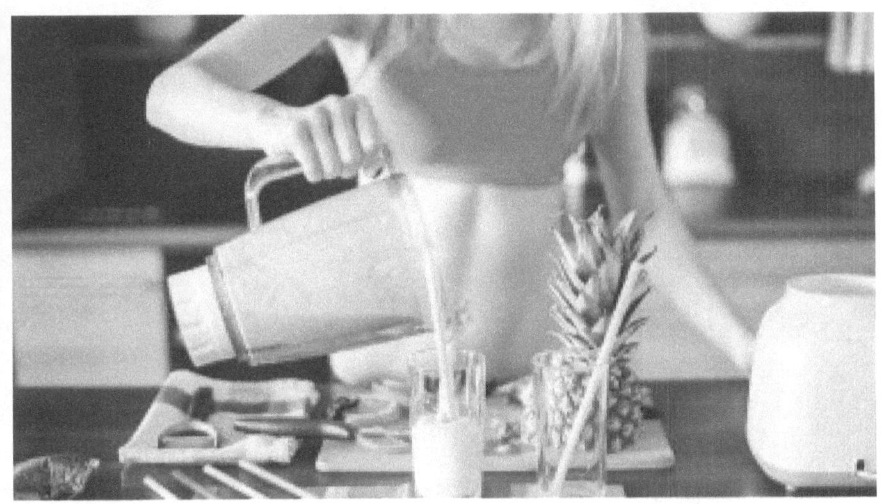

Unnecessary cuts in food intake, fasting, or quick useless diets lead to a drastic reduction in BMR. Many do this so that the body starts to burn its own energy supplies, most often to quickly lose weight. Those who think this method is effective are obviously not familiar with how metabolism works.

Water, the Liquid of Life

The speed of our metabolism depends on whether we are taking plenty of liquid. Drinking water before meal improves digestion. In this way, ferments responsible for digestion are diluted, so the absorption of nutrients and the elimination of toxins is increased. Whether hot or cold, water is essential.

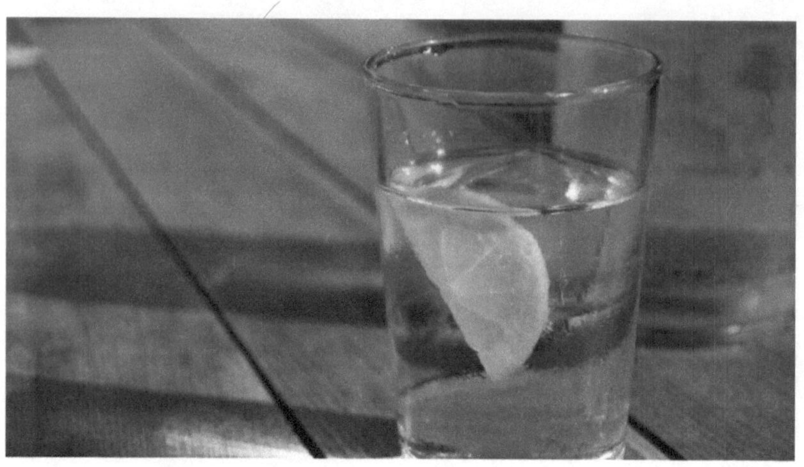

Warm water improves digestion and increases body temperature. The temperature difference should not be extreme, but it stimulates metabolism and initiates more energy to be burned. This cause-effect relationship keeps the optimal balance of caloric input and consumption.

Cold water decreases the body temperature and "forces it" to maintain a warm internal body system. This process requires additional energy, or increased calorie burning, and makes metabolism work at an accelerated pace.

Workout

Physical activity or the lack of it is another major factor that can affect slow metabolism. When we exercise, we build muscle mass and eliminate fatty deposits from the body. The more muscle groups we use, the body needs to replenish by producing more, while also consuming more energy. If you were active so far, a small change in the workout routine is all you need. Professional trainers recommend circular and strength training.

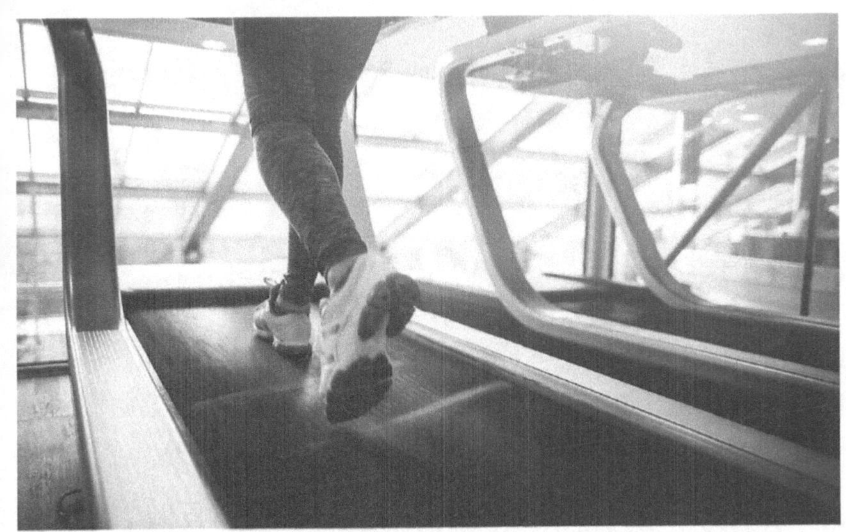

Every physical activity has some benefits for health. But what we advise is to change the intensity of exercise during a single training session. It can be achieved with circular training. Start slowly, and then suddenly boost the intensity of exercising, afterward, slow down again. This pace will help you speed up your metabolism in the long run.

As for people who haven't been exercising so far, in agreement with a professional trainer, they should opt for some easy training for a start, and monitor changes in their health. But, if you lack sufficient time for exercise, then it will be all right for you to walk. If possible, hike 2 to 3 kilometers in the fresh air, and lightly extend the route. Walk fast enough, so that you do not get too exhausted, and change the tempo every few minutes.

Chapter 4: Foods for Metabolism Boosting

There are foods to help you speed up your metabolism and free your organism from toxins that burden it and endanger your health. These are foods that abound in nutrients and are best consumed in unprocessed form. It is essential that you take each of these items along with other healthy foods.

For speeding up the metabolism, there is a "do's and don'ts" list of what you should eat or avoid. It is necessary to properly combine food groups so your digestive system won't get too burdened. This way, the organism can process all foods and extract the essential nutrients.

Integral or Whole Grain Cereals

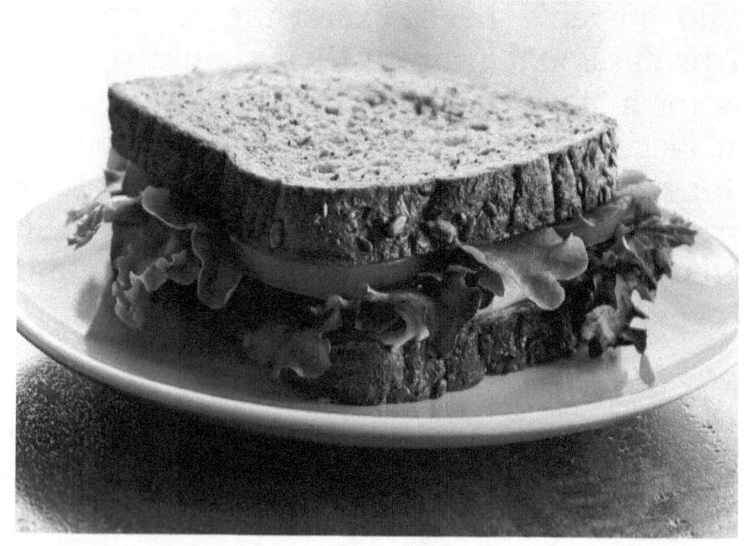

Integral cereals contain a handful of fibers and carbs which are recommended in daily nutrition. Eating whole grains will not only suppress appetite but will also stimulate digestion and eliminate toxins.

Whole grain foods have a copious amount of fibers and complex carbs that slowly disintegrate in our body. It takes more time for the body to digest these nutrients; it means that the energy is released gradually, and the active digestive system makes our metabolism work faster.

Every nutritionist will recommend you to consume whole grains for breakfast. After waking up in the morning, our body is most active because it has rested during the night. At that time, the activity of our digestive system is enhanced, and it can be involved in the digestion of fibers and complex carbs. These foods will provide energy for the whole day.

It is important to point out that you have to buy authentic cereals like buckwheat, barley, oats, spelt, etc. Not 5-minutes oatmeal or instant porridges with the addition of dried fruit, nut or chocolate aromas that you can find in every supermarket. These are full of unnecessary additives and sugars. Making your own whole grain meal won't take you too much time, and you'll know that's the real deal.

Coffee and Green Tea

Coffee is an ingredient rich in antioxidants, and if used in the recommended amount, has numerous benefits for our health and metabolism. It is a common fact that coffee contains caffeine, a natural stimulus that affects the central nervous system and speeds up metabolism. Some studies show that this acceleration goes up to 10% if we consume two cups of coffee without extras during the day.

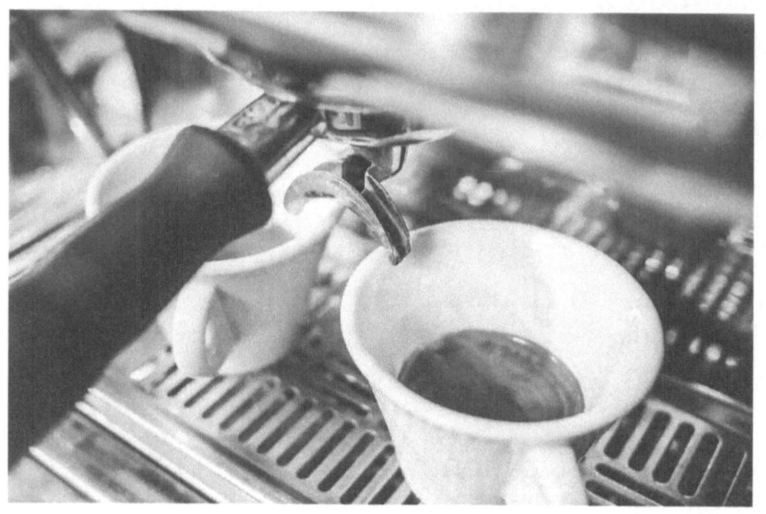

Three hours after just one cup of coffee, the metabolism is accelerating, and it comes to a thermogenic effect where the burning of lipids increases. Simply put, coffee increases the utilization of fats stored in the body. It will use them in the processes of obtaining and consuming energy required for the functioning of the body.

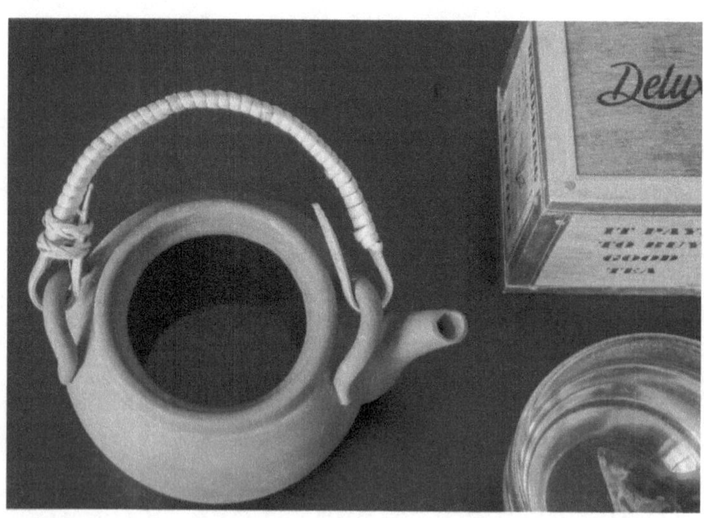

Besides coffee, it is desirable to have at least one cup of green tea on a daily basis. Its positive effect on the process of weight loss has been known for a long time. Antioxidants like catechins that is found in this tea have a similar influence on our body like caffeine.

Catechins are responsible for the gradual acceleration of our metabolism within 24 hours. Our body is stimulated to consume energy supplies from fat deposits, which leads to a healthy weight loss and detoxification of the body.

Spices and Herbs

Besides giving every dish a better taste, spices and fresh herbs have numerous positive effects on our health, which we are often unaware of. The addition of a variety of flavors can help digestion and boost metabolism.

Whether it's a sour like turmeric, hot as pepper and chili, or musky aroma like cinnamon, these ingredients contain elements that slightly increase the body temperature. In this way, they induce metabolism to start the process of fat burning, which represents supplies of unused energy. The spicy components stimulate the production of gall and stomach juices, which play an essential role in the digestion process.

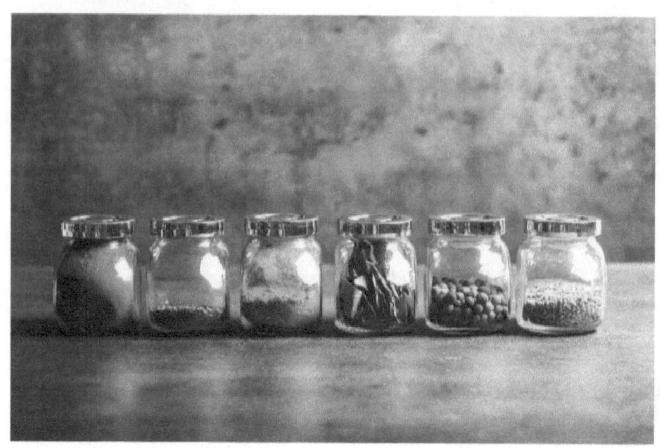

Organic substances found in aromatic herbs such as marjoram, parsley or oregano also help to burn fat and speed up metabolism. At the same time, they prevent the fast growth of the blood sugar level. Essential oils found in these fresh herbs stimulate the production of enzymes and make the process of food digestion more efficient.

Ginger has proved useful in the process of detoxification of the body. It enhances the elimination of toxins and prevents excessive carb absorption. Excess carbs are likely to result in new fat deposits and excessive weight gain ultimately.

Aromatic spices and herbs can be used every day, and there are no specific restrictions on their use. You should use them to the extent that they do not cause problems with bloating or gastric acid. You can add them to dishes, drinks, pastries or even a glass of water (cinnamon in combination with honey every day before breakfast is a score).

Citruses and Red Fruits

It is known that citrus fruits contain many antioxidants that are natural cleansers of the body. Flavonoids, one of the essential antioxidants, are especially useful for boosting metabolism. These microelements are quickly absorbed into the body, and then instantly secreted out of it. In this process, they bring out numerous toxins from the liver and gallbladder.

Regular consumption of orange, lemons, mandarin, limes or grapefruit will bring multiple benefits to your body. These are the foods you should eat fresh every day, in the form of juices, smoothies, cakes or fruit salads.

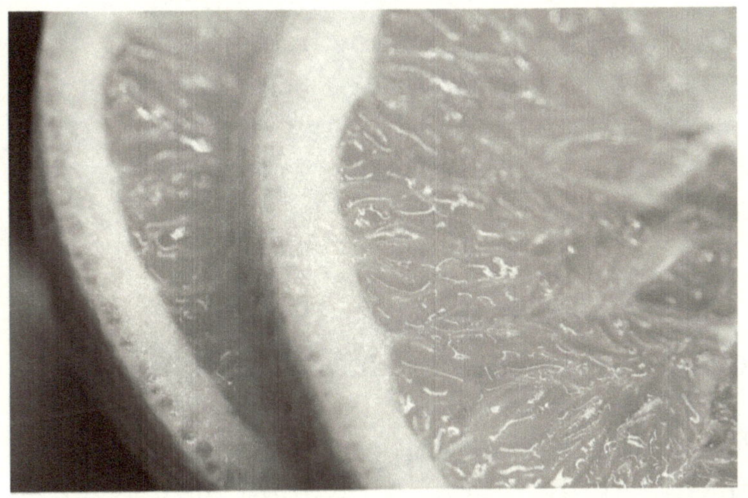

Also, red fruits like raspberries, blackberry and blueberries are rich in flavonoids too. These antioxidants prevent the body to deposit extra fat by limiting its absorption. Eating berries instead of processed candies and chocolate bars are good for staying slim, fit and healthy. Only one handful of red fruits per day is enough to trigger metabolism, and you will see the results in no time at all.

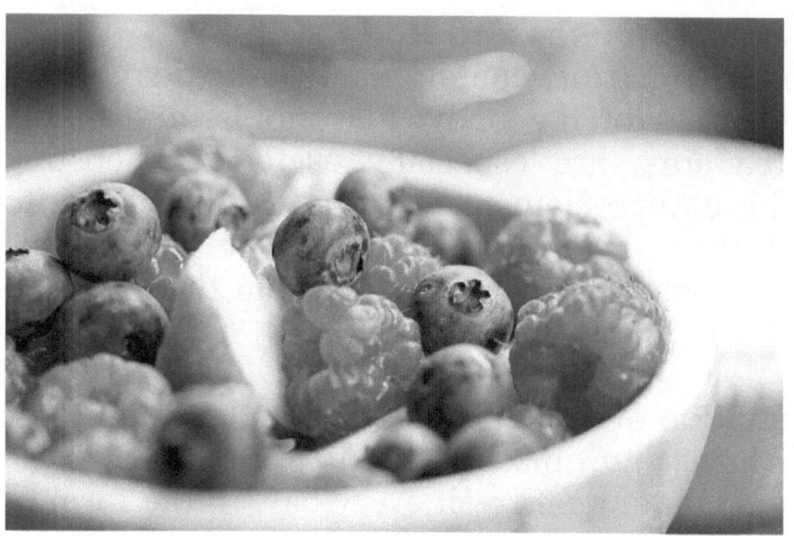

Thermal treatment of fruits is not recommended; besides losing nutrients, the concentration of sugar increases, which can lead to the appearance of excessive weight. However, from time to time it is not a bad idea to treat ourselves to dry fruits as a snack. These have plenty of fibers that are excellent cleaners of the bowels.

Seasonal Vegetables

Many foods are low in calories but are loaded with nutrients, and are an excellent way to speed up metabolism. Valuable minerals abound in this food group, so they should form a significant part of your daily menu. A brilliant choice is the veggies that contain plenty of water, such as cucumber, zucchini, or lettuce.

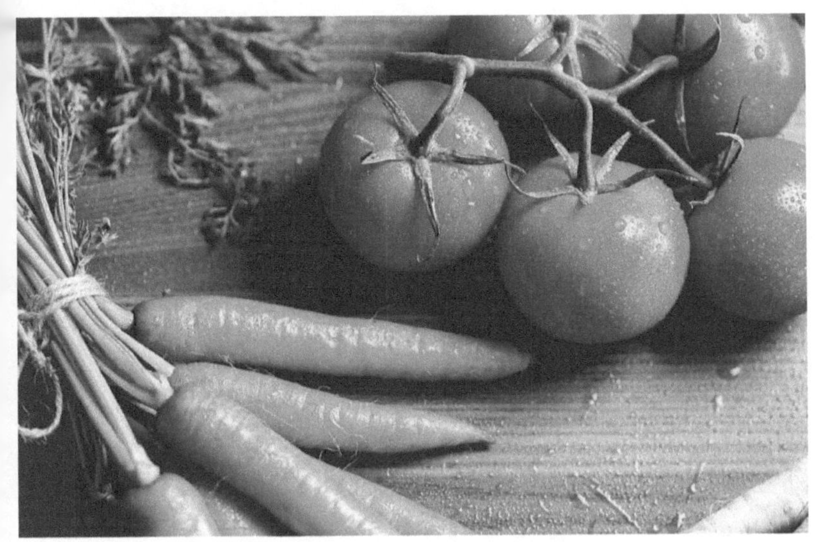

Digestion of this food is easy; the absorption of nutrients is on the maximal level, and what is best is that such vegetables contain so-called "negative calories." It doesn't mean that those ingredients have no calories because that is a myth. It only implies that some veggies have very low caloric value— they won't become fat deposits; our body even burns more energy to digest them.

For example, for the digestion of a mixed vegetable salad, the body has to spend a certain percentage of its energy reserves. If you replace just one part of the meal with a spicy salad of mixed veggies, the results will soon be evident. Fresh vegetables contain insoluble fiber that cleans the gastrointestinal tract. In the process of passing through our bowels, these fibers "collect" the waste that has accumulated in them and bring it out.

For metabolism boosting, we should eat more seasonal vegetables of a particular color. For example, in the summer we have to eat red, like tomatoes and peppers; in the spring, all sorts of cabbages and greens would do, while autumn and winter nutrition should be enriched with vegetables that provide more energy and heat the body, such as lentils, beans, potatoes, etc. We recommend you to consume raw vegetables or very lightly processed ones because, in this form, they contain less fat and organic sugars.

Common Mistakes We Make and How to Avoid Them

There are some rules we have to follow if we want to improve our digestion and keep the optimal metabolism speed. Even the healthiest foods won't have any effect if meals are incorrectly distributed and combined during the day. Sure, we can't follow all of them, but we could try to adhere to a couple of the essential ones:

1. Carbohydrates and animal proteins should not be consumed in the same meal. Although it is customary to eat potatoes or rice with meat, or bread with dishes like curry or stew, this is not recommended. In this combination, digestion is difficult, and gases and stomach cramps are inevitable.

2. Eating candies and fruits after an abundant main meal that is full of animal proteins complicate digestion, causing heartburn and decreased production of stomach acid.

3. Avoid mixing milk and dairy products with meat. Milk
    starts to clot when it reaches the stomach and slows
    the digestion of other foods. Proteins from meat take a
    long time to dilute so this will be real torture for your
    organism.

4. Vegetables and fruits should not be consumed in one
    meal. The time for digestion of these foods varies
    considerably. Because of the amount of sugar, the fruit
    begins to ferment, causing stomach problems. Pay
    attention in combining just fruit or veggies; mix only
    those of similar characteristics and tastes.

Chapter 5: Time to Detox

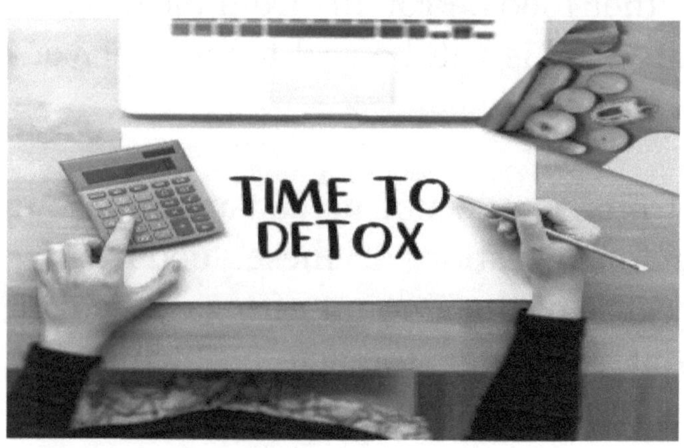

From time to time our body needs help getting rid of accumulated toxins. However, most often, different diets are used primarily to get rid of extra pounds.

Even those who are not overweight, it is useful to periodically have a fasting period to get rid of all the excess toxins in the body, especially after holidays with frequent overeating.

Detox is one of the most fashionable beauty trends. Cosmetics manufacturers produce detox creams, masks and cleansers, and, of course, they have an effect. But, as you know, beauty begins from the inside, and therefore a detox diet should be the first step in cleansing the body.

Like any other diet, detox diets have positive and negative points.

Many people really feel more energetic, lighter and generally better after doing a detox. Nutritionists explain that this happens for two reasons: the first is the legendary placebo effect, and the second is the lack of processed foods in the diet.

The reason why a detox diet improves the general condition of the body is because the individual starts getting proper nutrition. So, a healthy diet with enough protein, proper fat and fiber will definitely work just as well as, or most likely better than, popular detox programs. Keep this in mind before changing your diet for the purpose of losing weight or healing.

Organic Detox

This program slowly but surely will teach you not only to eat right, but also to live right. When consuming=natural products, the diet adjusts to having a good metabolism. And this is the key to good health and appearance.

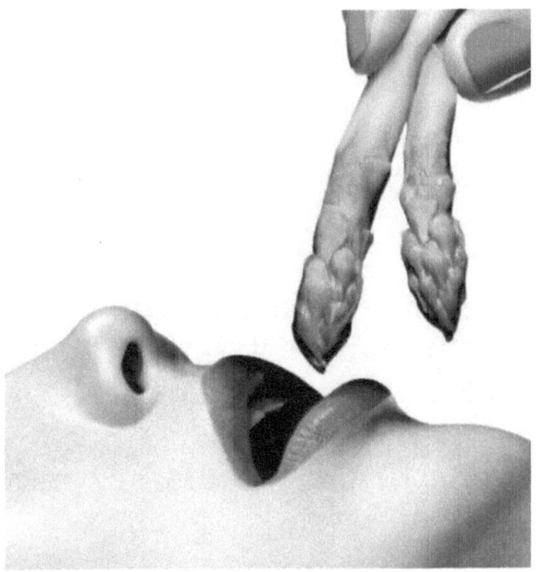

WHAT TO DO

- Exclude processed products saturated with growth hormones, pesticides, preservatives and other synthetic components.

- Switch to organic products, which can be found in special departments of grocery stores and markets.

- Limit the consumption of animal proteins (no more than 150 g of eggs, fish, lean steamed meat, dairy products and hard or goat cheese).

- Give up sugar for 15 days, and then reduce its consumption to once a week.

- Forget about "saturated" fatty acids: margarine, palm oil, fatty meat.

- Become accustomed to unsaturated fatty acids (olive, linseed, rapeseed oil, walnut oil and pumpkin seeds).

- Focus on green vegetables, plant sprouts, fruits, almonds, rice milk, brown rice, corn.

- Cook only with olive oil, and when buying choosing organic varieties.

- Clean the intestinal walls (the professional procedure of hydrocolonotherapy can replace the use of laxatives - 1 tablespoon of magnesium chloride in a glass of water).

- Take probiotics that restore intestinal flora and enzymes (sold in pharmacies).

- Saturate the body with oxygen, devoting 30 minutes a day to walks or jogging in the fresh air. An alternative to walking is using oxygen spray, which can be bought at any pharmacy.

- Visit a sauna, Turkish or Russian bath for the additional removal of toxins.

- Sign up for a draining or shiatsu massage.

- To drink pure spring water.

- Meet the body's need for vitamins, minerals and amino acids by taking supplements.

Two Week Menu

Immediately after waking:
A glass of warm water with the juice of half a lemon
Large glass of freshly squeezed vegetable juice

Breakfast:
Green tea with grated ginger and lemon
A slice of wheat bread with grated almonds or avocado puree
At 10 o'clock:
Vitamin C (ascorbic acid)

Lunch:
- Soup-puree of steamed vegetables
- Brown rice and steamed vegetables with olive oil

At 4 o'clock:
Fruit puree with a couple of nuts and a few almonds

Supper:
- Soup-puree of steamed vegetables

- Fatty fish of the red or white variety three times a week, white meat twice a week, two eggs once a week, goat cheese or mozzarella once a week.

- Steamed vegetables

Chapter 6: Detox Diet - General Cleaning of the Body for 10 Days!

10-Day Detox Diet - this is a nutrition system that is primarily aimed at getting rid of toxins, and hence the improvement of the whole body.

The main goal of a detox diet is to rid the body of toxins and make it healthier, so the program is not only limited to the principles of nutrition. It is recommended you supplement the diet with a course of massage, calm physical activity (yoga, walking, or swimming), saunas or baths.

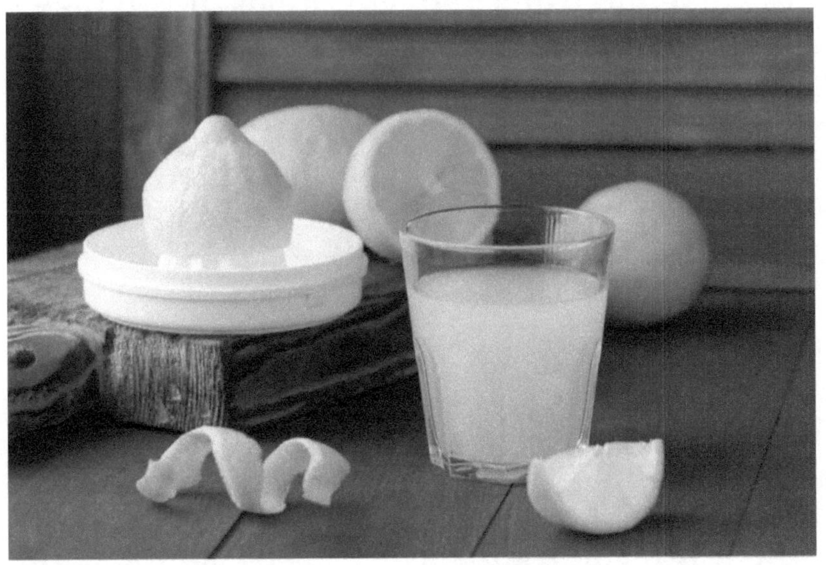

Observe the Rules

Detoxification is the removal of toxins and waste products from the body. However, this process requires following a number of rules that will make detoxification as effective and safe as possible. It is better not to try a detox diet if you're only doing it half way, and be sure to consult your doctor! Detox programs are not good for everyone; teenagers, people with gastrointestinal diseases (gastritis, ulcers), and athletes on the eve of the competition should not follow this kind of diet.

For proper and gentle cleansing of the body is important to prepare well. If you ate sweets and fat yesterday, and today decide to limit yourself to fruits and light foods, it is unlikely that you will feel good. The body will require more high-calorie food, as you may get a headache due to the sharp drop in blood sugar. Therefore, for a soft transition to the detox menu, we advise you to start preparing a month before the planned program. To do this, you should do the following:

* Completely eliminate alcohol;

* Gradually reduce and completely stop eating fried and fatty foods, flour, sweets, and processed products;

* Plan to eat the last meal of the day at least 3 hours before bedtime;

* Reduce serving sizes and eat often (every 4 hours);

* Include as many vegetables and fresh herbs as possible in your meals;

* A week before the detox diet switch to lighter foods, and it is best to completely cut out meat. The basis of your diet at this time will be grains, vegetables, fruits, low-fat cheese, and dairy products.

In addition to preparing, it is important to choose the right time to purify the body. The best season for detoxification is the beginning of autumn or spring. At this time, the body is much more willing to part with the accumulated toxins, and therefore you can easily adopt the diet with greater efficiency. Do not abruptly start a detox program after the Christmas holidays. Do not forget that the body needs preparation for a soft transition to a new diet.

Another trick to planning a detox diet is to choose a 10-day cleansing period when you are on vacation. Calmness, relaxation and rest will only enhance the effects of detoxification. Besides, you will have more time for additional procedures, walks and sports. If you can not synchronize the diet with a vacation, then try to choose a time that is not particularly stressful, for example, during the replacement of another employee.

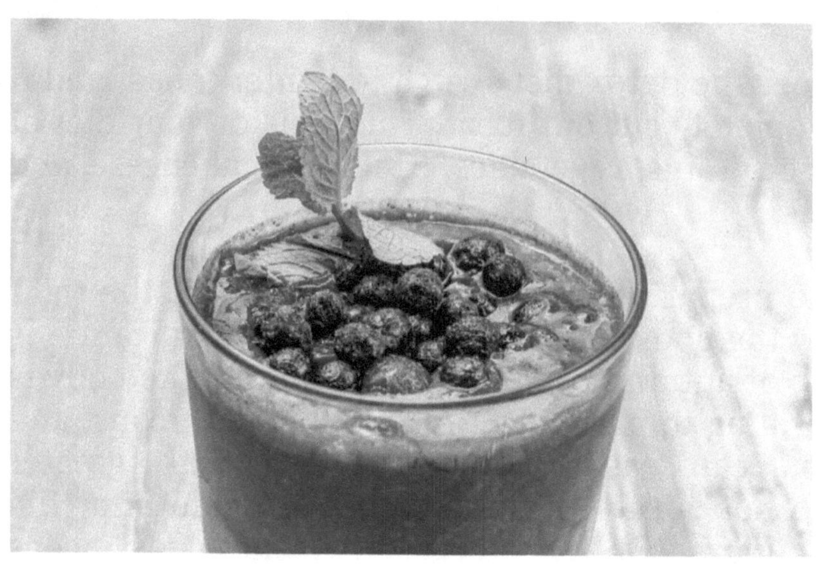

Choose the Duration of the Diet: 3, 5, 7 or 10 Days?

If you have never performed a detoxification of the body, you should start with the easier option of 3 days. A detox diet for 3 days at home can be followed easily enough; it can be planned for the weekend. This procedure will prepare you for subsequent cycles of detoxification. At the same time, do not forget about reasonable preparation, and you will see positive results such as improved health and weight loss even after a brief cleansing program.

If you care about your health and have already conducted a course of cleansing the body, you can try a 5 or 7-day detoxification. With a 5-7-day program, the effects will be much greater: your metabolism will be accelerated, you will feel lighter, the size of your stomach will decrease, and habits of proper nutrition will begin to form.

If you are already familiar with the principles of proper nutrition, you can proceed to a more complex level – a diet for 10 days. A 10-day detox will not only improve the functioning of your gastrointestinal tract, but also cleanse the blood and normalize cholesterol levels.

During the program, you will lose about 6-7 kilograms. Doing a detox diet for longer than 10 days is not recommended, as this diet is not nutritionally balanced – it is aimed at removing toxins from the body. After the end of the diet, you can carefully return to a normal, healthy diet. To maintain the effects, you should avoid unhealthy eating habits. It is recommended to do a detox once every 6 months.

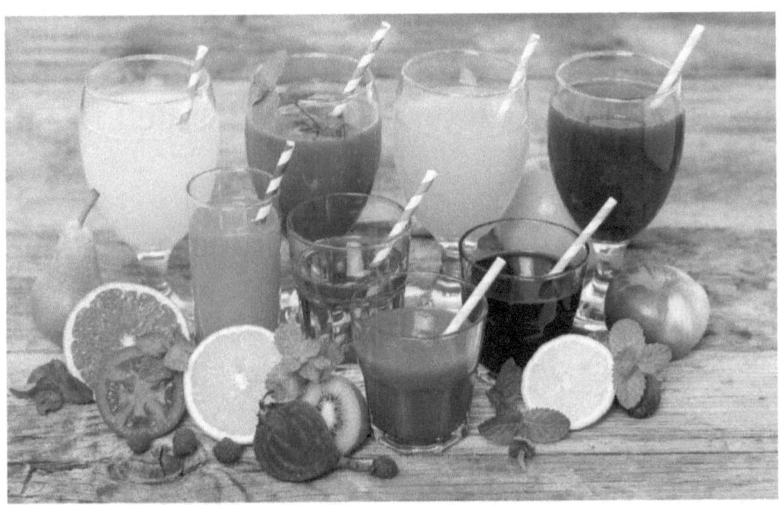

Menu for 3-Day Detox

For those who cannot tolerate long diets but want to take care of their health, it is easy to spend 3 days cleansing the body. The menu for each of the 3 days is the same, which allows for worry-free meal planning.

Breakfast: The day begins with a detox lemonade, which is not difficult to prepare. In a glass of warm water squeeze the juice of half a lemon. Add crushed or finely grated ginger root (a small piece). Half an hour after drinking the lemonade you can prepare the main breakfast meal, a fresh fruit or vegetable smoothie. Choose products that suit your tastes and budget. For purification, a good choice is green apples, cabbage, spinach, celery, and cucumber. You can also add lemon juice.

Lunch: For lunch prepare a special detox soup. It's not quite soup in the traditional sense of the word; it is very easy, low calorie, and all the ingredients are just cooked. Ingredients: 4 glasses of water, 2 small zucchini (cut into cubes), 2 tomatoes, 3 celery stalks, 1 carrot, 1 cup of chopped cabbage. For seasoning add garlic, black pepper, oregano, and parsley. Put all the vegetables in a pot with the water and cook for about 30 minutes. This soup will be enough for lunch for all 3 days.

Afternoon snack: Salad made of spinach, Chinese cabbage and boiled chicken breast in equal proportions. You can add cucumber, carrot, tomato, and a small amount of nuts to taste. You can also add parsley, onion and a small amount of lemon juice.

Supper: Make another smoothie of fresh vegetables and / or fruit to your taste. Shortly before you go to sleep, you can drink a glass of chamomile tea to calm down and sleep more soundly, especially if you are not used to falling asleep on an empty stomach.

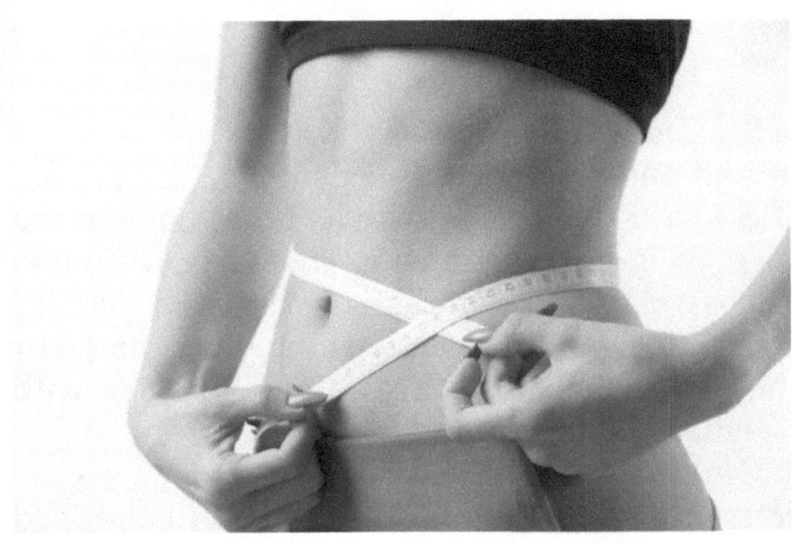

Detox Diet for 5 Days

Breakfast: Start each day with home-made oatmeal made from one cup of oat flakes and 4 cups of water or with a green smoothie of your choice (you can use any green fruits or vegetables, add lemon, ginger, and spices to taste). In the oatmeal, you can also add berries and sweet spices like cinnamon or vanilla, and you can sweeten it with one teaspoon of honey if you wish.

Day 1:
Lunch: Fresh Kale Salad
Mix chopped kale with fresh carrot, a few slices of red onion, and 2 tablespoons of pumpkin seeds. Season with salt, pepper, olive oil, and lemon juice.
Dinner: Colorful Plate
Make a salad of chopped spinach, tomato, pepper, ¼ cup ground cinnamon and fresh herbs such as basil and parsley. You can add pumpkin or sunflower seeds if you wish. Season it with apple cider vinegar, olive oil, and salt. Feel free to substitute or add other types of vegetables that are seasonally accessible.

Day 2:
Lunch: Paprika Stuffed with Quinoa
Cut a pepper in half and remove the seeds. Place the pepper halves on a foil-coated tray, season with salt and bake in the oven until the pepper is soft. Meanwhile, in a large bowl mix boiled black beans, chopped tomatoes, chili, and parsley leaves. Add some olive oil, salt, and lemon juice and stir together. Fill the pepper halves with stuffing and serve with fresh cabbage-salad.
Dinner: Carrot 'Omelet' and Boiled Broccoli
Add young onions to heated olive oil, and then add chopped carrot. After two minutes, add tomatoes, chopped onion, spinach, and spices (saffron or turmeric will give this dish a real omelet color). Serve with steamed broccoli drizzled with lemon juice.

Day 3:
Lunch: Lentil Stew
Cook lentils in plenty of water. After 20 minutes of cooking, stir until they completely absorb the water. Finally, when the dish thickens, add oregano, garlic, parsley, and sea salt.
Dinner: Grilled Zucchini with Tofu and Fresh Cabbage Salad
Grill zucchini on medium heat. Serve with tofu cheese slices and cabbage salad that is seasoned with olive oil, lemon juice, salt, and pepper.

Day 4:
Lunch: Polenta Sticks and Tomato Salad
Pour cornmeal into boiling water and cook until it thickens. Remove from the stove, add chopped spinach, mix and spread the mixture on an oiled tray. Cut cooled polenta into sticks and serve with a salad of fresh tomato, parsley, olive oil, salt, and pepper.
Dinner: Quinoa Bean Dish

Mix cooked quinoa and beans, and add chopped bell pepper, tomato, and spring onion, and season with a handful of fresh herbs.

<u>Day 5</u>:
Lunch: Pumpkin Stew
Soak the beans overnight to rest. Stir-fry chopped pumpkin in olive oil, and add 2 cups of water. When it steams a bit, add beans and cook on low heat. When the beans are almost cooked, add salt and cook for another 15-30 minutes. Turn off the heat and leave for a few minutes. Sprinkle with chopped fresh parsley leaves before serving.
Dinner: Fresh Kale Salad
Have the same dish as the lunch from Day 1.

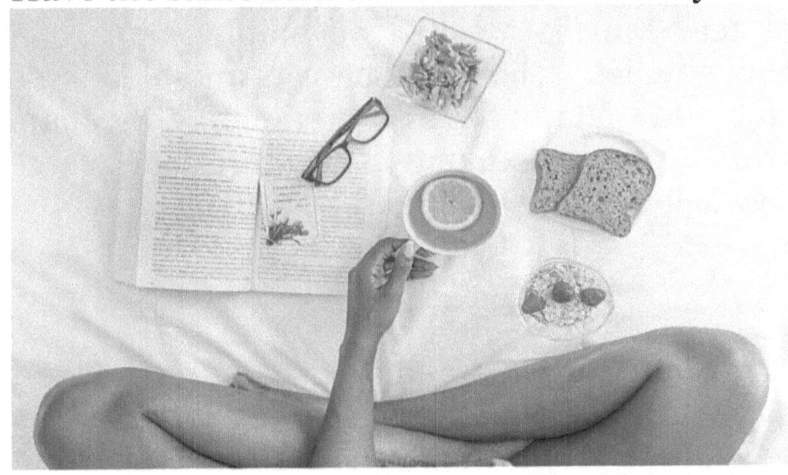

Detox Diet for 7 and 10 Days

For the 7-and 10-day detox programs, the menu is about the same; the only difference is how long you follow the diet for. Do not forget, if you originally planned a 10-day course, but then stopped after 7 days, it is important to exit the diet correctly. Below is a detox program for 7 days, and the menu is a little more satisfying than for a 3-day diet.

Day 1

Start the day with a glass of warm water with a small amount of lemon juice. Half an hour later eat a basic *Breakfast*: Whole grain bread with the flesh of an avocado and ginger tea. *Lunch*: Boiled rice without salt and a selection of vegetables of your choice (except any starchy options). Afternoon snack: Green apple. *Dinner*: Fresh vegetables and two hard-boiled eggs, combined to make the salad, and seasoned with lemon juice.

Day 2

A glass of warm water with 0.5 tsp honey, half an hour after waking up. *Breakfast*: Vegetable salad without dressing (you can use a little lemon juice), 1 slice of whole grain bread, mint or herbal tea. *Lunch*: Mashed vegetable soup (boil cabbage, zucchini, spinach, celery, and carrots and blend in a blender). Do not add salt, butter, or cream to this soup. *Snack*: Any fruit (except bananas). *Dinner*: The same vegetable and egg salad from Day 1, except you can add low-fat cheese.

Day 3

Water with orange juice upon waking. *Breakfast:* Low-fat cottage cheese, green apple and any herbal tea. *Lunch:* Any easy vegetable soup. During the day, grab a grapefruit. *Dinner:* Treat yourself to boiled or baked fish with a vegetable salad.

Day 4

Water with lemon juice upon waking. *Breakfast*: Fruit salad. *Lunch*: Pureed vegetable soup. *Afternoon snack*: A small number of nuts (7-10 pieces). *Dinner*: Salad with boiled chicken breast and vegetables.

Day 5

Water with orange juice upon waking. *Breakfast:* Cottage cheese and any fruit. *Lunch:* Pumpkin soup. *Afternoon snack*: Two kiwi fruit. *Dinner*: Boiled fish and salad.

Day 6
On an empty stomach, drink some water with lemon. *Breakfast:* Eat your favorite fruit. *Lunch:* Eat a portion of boiled rice with vegetables. *Afternoon snack:* Have a cup of yogurt. *Dinner*: Boiled chicken and vegetables.

Day 7
This is the final day, so follow the same menu as Day 1.
If you plan to continue, a detox diet with menu for 10 days will look like this:

Day 7
Glass of water with lemon juice. *Breakfast:* Bread with avocado, tomato, and ginger / herbal tea. *Lunch:* Green soup. *Afternoon snack:* Baked apple. *Dinner*: Grilled/steamed vegetables. Before going to bed, drink a decoction of prunes.

Day 8
Glass of water with honey. *Breakfast*: Cabbage salad and carrots. *Lunch:* Broccoli/Chinese cabbage soup. *Afternoon snack*: Fruit or smoothie. *Dinner*: Vegetable stew.

Day 9
In the morning drink some water with lemon. *Breakfast*: Cucumbers, cottage cheese, and parsley. *Lunch:* Vegetable soup. *Snack*: An orange/grapefruit. *Dinner*: Chicken fillet and salad with fresh vegetables.

Day 10
Repeat the menu from Day 1.

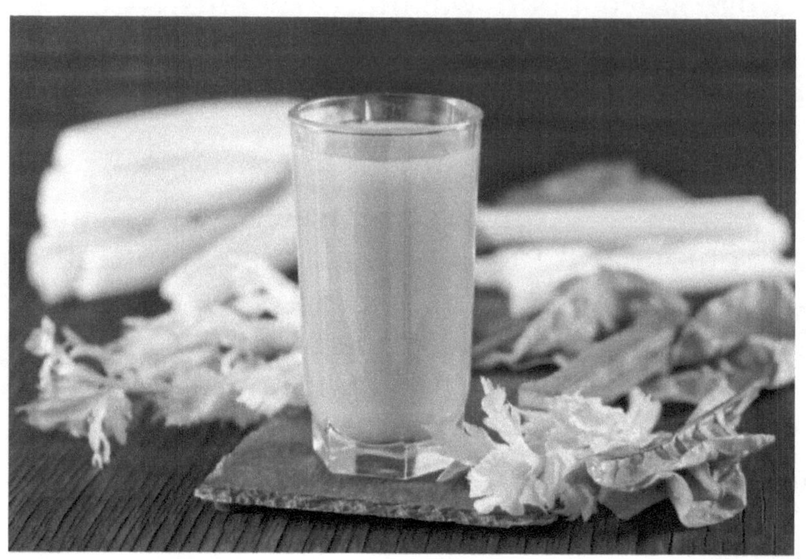

The detox program (the menu for a week) is variable. For example, you can replace one fruit with another, or replace chicken breast with low-fat fish. The menu stays basically the same, just with different combinations of ingredients so the meals do not become boring.

Chapter 7: Does a Detox Diet Really Cleanse the Body?

So, now let's talk about how detox diets work, why they can be harmful, and how to cleanse your body while maintaining your sanity.

Why are we talking about sanity? Firstly, because a famous magazine found out through the course of conducting a study that one American woman in twenty would rather lose an arm or leg than gain weight. The residents of the United States are not fundamentally different from the millions of other reasonable and educated women around the world who are obsessed with diets. For example, detox diets are now fashionable and are considered a great way to quickly eliminate extra pounds and dull complexion.

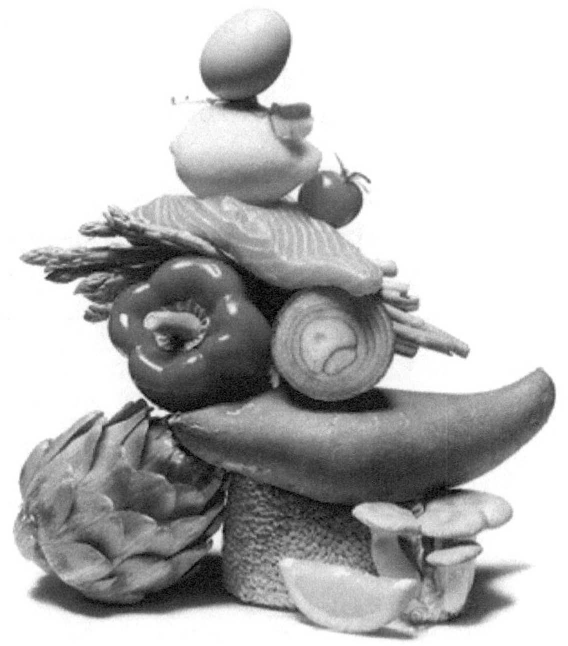

The idea itself looks great: You eat little, drink as much liquid as you can (and therefore spend the best part of the day on the toilet), and invisible toxins quickly leave the body. In reality, everything is not so great.

What is the Danger?

The concept of fasting days where people lean on a particular product or drink is not new. Fasting trends began in the 1930s, with the popular grapefruit diet. Over the years, the formula has not changed: those who want to lose weight are encouraged to reduce their calorie intake to a minimum and add some magical ingredient with incredible fat burning properties - cayenne pepper, or vinegar, or something equally tasty.

There is no scientific justification behind this advice - the consumption of only one product during the week (especially lettuce grown on chemical fertilizers) cannot cleanse the body of certain "toxins". And, by the way, our body has systems in place to process and eliminate toxins: the kidneys and the liver, not the shortest part of the digestive tract.

But what is most unpleasant in detox diets? The various drugs and supplements that promise to cleanse the body most often are not approved as a medicine or food product, and their effects on the body have simply not been studied. At best, they are a common diuretic that flushes out potassium and other vital elements. In all honesty, many people sacrifice both sodium and potassium for impressive results.

On such a "diet", the body loses only water, and only for a short time. When the person goes back to their normal eating habits, the weight that was lost quickly returns. If the weight continues to decrease, it means that the muscles, not the fat, are depleted. Without a sufficient amount of protein (and liquid), the human body begins to produce the necessary energy by using its own muscle tissue.

Do not worry, you say? Do not lie to yourself. Our muscles are a calorie-burning mechanism built into the body. It is in the muscle tissue that cupcakes and sausages are processed. And the more muscle you have, the more calories you burn, even while just sitting around. But the less you eat, the slower your metabolism.

After a couple of days on a low-calorie diet, the metabolism is significantly inhibited. The body thinks that there is a shortage of food and panics. The consumption of calories is reduced in order to maintain the maximum functioning of the body in difficult times.

Effects

Everyone understands that detox diets cause one to eat less and thereby reduce caloric intake. But studies have found a less obvious fact: After just a few days on a strict diet (when the daily caloric intake does not exceed 1200 kcal), the human body stops producing the most important IGF-1 protein (an insulin-like growth factor) and reduces the production of thyroid hormones, insulin and some other hormones. Over time, this leads to problems of various kinds - from bones becoming brittle to the development of mental disorders.

Some individuals, suspecting possible harm from diets, prefer gentle tactics - fasting every other day. This kind of nutritional plan, as shown by a clinical study, is really good for people suffering from obesity, but not very effective for those who want to get rid of just a couple of kilograms. But the quality of life is noticeably affected. People who sharply limit caloric intake are easily recognizable by their irritability due to hunger, complaints of constant fatigue and confessions that even thinking about sex is disgusting. And what is the use of a beautiful body if the only thing you want is to go to bed?

Expert Opinion

In addition to popular opinions on any diet, including detox diets ("one girl ate only vegetable soup and got rid of all her diseases and lost 20 kg, let's do the same thing"), there is also the necessity of medical evaluation.

The overwhelming majority of detox systems offer approximately the same diet: two types of berries and two types of vegetable juices and liquid cream soup every day. However, from a medical point of view, to get rid of toxins, you need to drink more water, exclude fast food and consume solid foods containing fiber. The body should receive all the elements it needs comprehensively. Depriving yourself of any one of these disrupts an important biochemical balance. And the motto of the detox movement itself - minus 10 kg in 21 days - is a crime in terms of the physiological processes of the human body.

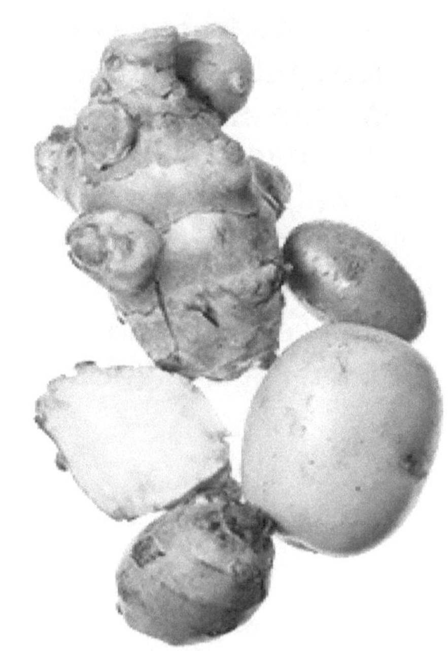

The rapid weight loss associated with the strict restriction of calories puts the body under great stress and does not normalize metabolic processes. Therefore, after abandoning the diet, the person will inevitably gain weight, and already against the background of problems in the gastrointestinal tract! For people who are controlling their weight, two or three fasting days per month are enough - when a person eats lighter and lower-calorie foods to help speed up metabolic processes and, as a result, gets rid of unnecessary toxins.

I also want to address hydrocolonotherapy, which is often recommended to supplement detox diets. Intestinal bacteria are extremely important for digestion, and it is not worth interfering with their environment without good reason. It is very easy to cause damage, which will lead to serious diseases of the gastrointestinal tract. Therefore, my main advice is to remember that the time-tested way to beauty, health and normal weight is a balanced diet, adequate physical activity and healthy sleep, at least six to eight hours a night.

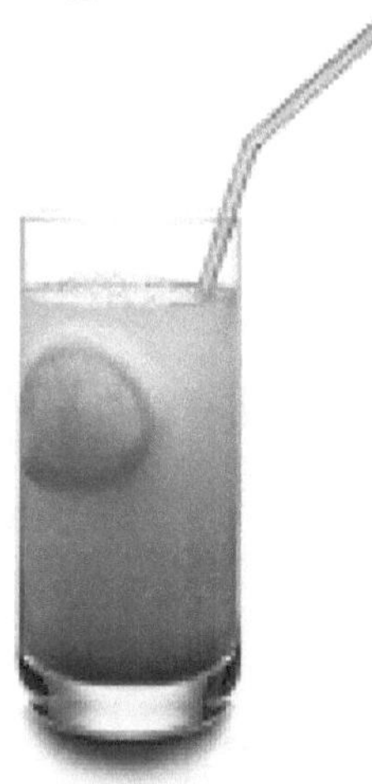

Do you believe in miraculous liquid diets? There is no magic in them; if you eat only a minimum of calories and a hiccup-inducing cocktail, you really lose weight. And health along with it.

Healthy Diet

Fasting diets may be helpful. Most people consume more calories than they need, overloading the liver and kidneys. However, a sensible diet not only gives the digestive system the necessary rest, but also saves a person from the influence of the main health-damaging factors: alcohol, excess sugar and saturated fat. Pay attention to the word "reasonable".

A proper cleansing diet should provide the right number of calories (this varies with each person depending on weight and age, but on average ranges from 1200 to 1800 kcal per day) and contain all the important trace elements, fiber and protein.

For example, a diet designed for a woman with a height of 160–165 cm and a weight of 52–56 kg (if your indicators differ, you will need to adjust upwards or downwards) suggests eating about 1500 kcal per day. In order to start losing weight and improve your health, you need to adhere to these requirements for 3 days.

To avoid surges in blood sugar and mood swings, you need to eat quite often — every 4 hours — and drinking enough water, decaffeinated tea, or herbal infusions. And then no nasty cocktails, bouts of fatigue and irritation!

DIET MENU
Breakfast
• 200 ml of non-carbonated water with freshly squeezed lemon juice
• An omelette made from three egg whites with fresh herbs (for example, basil or oregano), 1 tbsp. salsa and 1 slice of whole wheat toast or 1 cup of oatmeal with a handful of blueberries or 2 tsp. nuts
• 200 ml of decaffeinated green or herbal tea

Snack
• Apple with 1 tsp. natural peanut butter or 1/3 cup of trail mix (nuts and dried fruit)

Dinner
• 2 handfuls of fresh spinach or a mixture of spinach and kale, seasoned with lemon or orange juice

or 200 g of green asparagus with 1 tsp. olive oil, a clove of garlic and 1 tsp. lemon juice
• 120 g of baked, stewed or grilled salmon or seasoned chicken
• 100 g steamed green beans
• 200 ml of decaffeinated green or herbal tea
• 4 pecans

Snack
• ½ baked sweet potato or orange / grapefruit
• 120 ml of natural yogurt

Supper
• A large plate of spinach or romaine salad with fresh tomatoes, peppers, carrots, onions, and cucumbers, seasoned with 1 tsp. olive oil and 1 tsp. lemon juice
• 120 g chicken, baked or grilled, seasoned
• ½ cup brown rice, bulgur or quinoa
• 200 ml of decaffeinated green or herbal tea

Snack
• 1 cup blueberries or ½ glass pomegranate seeds
• 120 ml of natural yoghurt or soft curd cheese
There is so much fiber in asparagus that there is no better way to lose weight.
Red pepper is not only the most beautiful pepper but also the richest in antioxidants.
If you can't imagine life without sweets, pay attention to the yam - the perfect choice for a sensible dessert fan.

Chapter 8: The Easy Way to Live Without Diets is Up to You

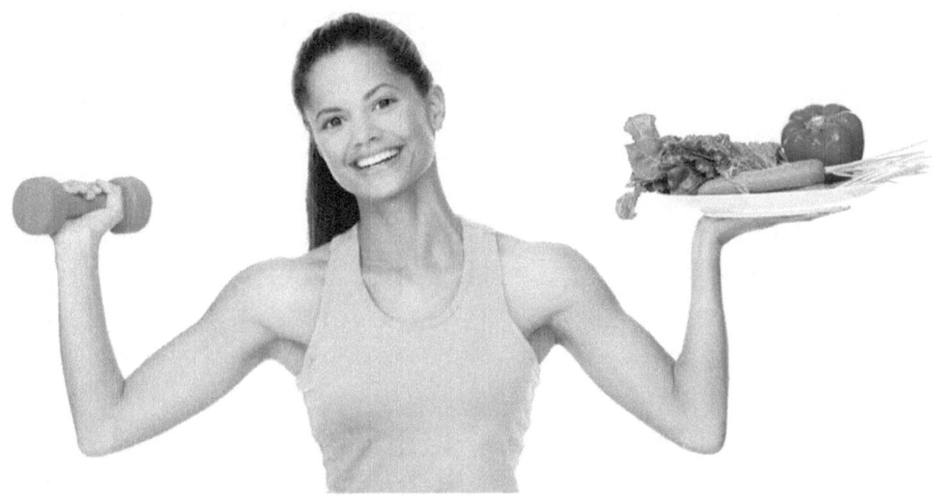

Anyone is overweight, or believes themselves to be, knows that there is a great variety of different diets, as well as nutritionists who make a name for themselves and make a lot of money promoting a particular nutrition system. It has long been observed that people who are prone to gaining extra weight, no matter what diets they try or how much they exercise, sooner or later they return to their previous weight, or even exceed it. On the other hand, there is a sufficient number of people who can eat whatever they want but still remain slim.

Perhaps the key to solving this problem is hidden in our psyche? After all, positive thinking and having a good mood allows you to break free from stereotypes in your thinking.

First of all, listen to your body. After all, we are all different. Everyone has a different constitution, metabolism, blood type, living conditions, habits and cravings. Perhaps you are not overweight. Or maybe your excess weight is only a myth created by the modern fashion industry. If, nevertheless, you decide that extra weight is holding you back, before you start a futile struggle with your weight, you need to change your mental attitude. Otherwise, you are doomed to experiencing temporary short-term success.

Pay attention to animals. Obesity is never observed in wild animals. But among domestic animals, especially dogs and cats, it is often possible to see overweight pets, just like among their masters.

Perhaps you should observe animals, having had their fill, bury the remains of their food for the future. That is, they know when to stop. And to maintain normal weight, they do not turn to a nutritionist and do not diet. Of course, there are periods of lack of food in nature when animals lose weight, and periods of plenty. But obese individuals in the wild do not exist.

So, an easy way to live without diets is to get rid of the stereotypes imposed on us. After all, animals do not think about calories. They absorb as much of their favorite and tasty food as they want and at the same time do not gain weight.

The formula for a happy life without diets is to eat your favorite food when you want and as much as you want, without restrictions, diets and exhausting workouts, while maintaining a normal, comfortable weight and living in harmony with each other. But one should distinguish between the concept of satiation and the concept of overeating. Overeating is a serious, fatal disease, and it deprives us of self-respect. Not a single living organism, except for rational people and animals tamed by man, suffers from overeating. This must be realized clearly: eat everything you want to full satiation, but not to the extent of overeating!

Pleasure from tasty food is granted to a person so they can support life, and not to disfigure their body, spoil their health, significantly deteriorate their quality of life, cause pity and contempt to others, and thus cause them to disrespect themselves.

Obesity is not only a deadly disease, but also an insidious one. After all, it occurs gradually and imperceptibly.

Many may argue that we should eat as much as we want - hence the extra weight. But think again about animals. They also eat as much as they want, but what they want to eat is exactly enough to maintain a healthy lifestyle. It turns out that the only intelligent species on earth is man is more stupid than animals.

Any diet turns the pleasant experience of enjoying food into a real nightmare. Firstly, you are already unhappy that you will have to limit yourself, but when it is time to eat, you are also forbidden to eat everything that you love - which also denies you pleasure. And how often do those practicing diets break down? And how long after stopping the diet was it possible to keep the weight from being gained back? Usually, it comes back in even larger quantities.

The main idea of an easy way to live without diets is really not to diet. Don't make getting rid of excess weight your goal, but rather a full life, where you can enjoy your reflection in the mirror. Your energy will overwhelm you, and eating high-quality food will bring you real pleasure.

The main thing is to create motivation and a corresponding emotional mood. Then you can start feeling positive emotions by reading this book. After all, the first step to a new life has already been taken.

Keep in mind children. They are not forced to eat bitter, salty, or spicy. After all, nature itself has instilled in our consciousness an instinctive concept of useful and harmful food. From birth, children are endowed with this knowledge - it is impossible to eat bitter. And with perseverance, we continue to retrain our instincts and impose harmful behavioral stereotypes, which subsequently lead to a catastrophe.

Another stereotype is that excessive consumption of food leads to excess weight. In fact, you should blame the volume of food itself and its quality. When we eat food that is unhealthy, we deprive the body of nutrition. As a result, we eat a lot while trying to satisfy an insatiable hunger, and we stretch the stomach. In this case the benefits are minimal and the harm is enormous.

Isn't it easier to look at whole history of mankind and remember our heritage? After all, until recently, people lived without diets and nutritionists. At the same time, they managed to survive in a variety of adverse conditions and survive to this day as a species. At the same time, obesity has never been as big a problem as it is today. It is clear that this is connected to both our modern, unhealthy way of life and with the consumption of refined, processed foods which are harmful and do not contain any nutritional value.

Let's go back to the animals. Every owner of a dog or cat knows that there are cases when they smell some kind of food which in our opinion is harmless, yet they do not touch it. They have the innate ability to recognize toxins.

Remember how hard it is to make a child eat when he does not want it. Nature has taken care to instill in us a wonderful indicator of the need to replenish our life forces - hunger. No living creatures, except an adult person, will touch food without feeling hungry. This is due to physical hunger, which causes our appetite, making us so pleased to eat. No wonder we express this wish: Enjoy your meal. After all, when we lose our appetite due to illness, then we do not get pleasure from food.

Another natural instinct is if you eat more than expected, you can literally vomit. That is, the body gets rid of excess food. But we persistently stretch our stomachs from childhood and teach them to absorb ever larger amounts of food. The less useful the food, the more is required for satiation and the more toxins arise when it is processed. And this excess results in fat.

Some persons say they don't eat much and only get fat from the water. But let's remember the prisoners of concentration camps or the hungry people of Africa. Neither hormonal peculiarities nor a slow metabolism help them gain weight. There are no fat ones.

We instinctively feel exactly what nutrients we lack. Remember how pregnant women crave certain foods. Their body signals the lack of certain elements for the proper development of the fetus. Children have the same ability. But through bad habits, we continue to destroy the instincts given to us by nature, including forcing children to eat when they refuse.

What is your optimal weight? How can you determine it without a scale and complex calculations? The answer is very simple: You should like your reflection in a bathing suit. But here again the stereotypes imposed by modern ideals of beauty come into play. Again, let us turn to animals: In the season of abundance they gain a little weight, which is stored in the winter or in the drought season. This allows them to survive.

Given the negative impact of mass media propaganda, most consider their normal weight to be overweight. Remember - the normal weight for you is one at which you feel comfortable and have no health problems. It is different for each individual.

So, should you throw away your scale? Of course not. By making changes in your mind and starting to eat right, you will inevitably start to lose weight. However, this does not happen abruptly, but gradually. Therefore, periodically weighing yourself at the same time (in the morning on an empty stomach) will confirm the positive feeling of weight loss and give you enthusiasm. It is useful to record the results and even draw a graph of your weight loss. Visual progress recorded on paper will give you inspiration.

Get rid of the imposed opinion that the most harmful food is that which is the most delicious. After all, advertising, driven by business, provides us with false information.

In fact, the most delicious food is the food that is most useful. Remember your feelings when you first tried alcohol or cigarettes. Not only was it unpleasant, but also caused nausea and vomiting. The body signaled to you that it was poison. But we persistently teach ourselves to absorb poisons.

Similarly, different cultures like certain tastes to which they are accustomed. So, Asians cannot live without rice, Italians without pasta, and Slavs without bread and potatoes. But keep in mind that your body will most accurately tell you what is most useful for you. The main thing is, do not ignore your body's requests and everything will work out for you.

Conclusion

The excessive weight usually leads to obesity. Further, it is the cause of many health problems. Accelerating metabolism stimulates many changes in the body that will result in reduced fat deposits. If you just put healthy ingredients on the everyday menu, and you do not give up junk and processed food, you won't have any benefits.

The temporary detox diet is not a strenuous regime. The occasional change in nutrition should be understood as a way of life that will suit everyone. So we have to give our body a little push from time to time. The occasional detoxification of the organism will have a positive impact on overall health. It may seem like too much of renunciation, but if you look at it in the long run, it will improve your health and the quality of life.

But before you get rid of excess weight, you need to understand the reason why you have gained weight. If there are no diseases that are contributing to your obesity, then you just need to pull yourself together and get the proper nutrition in combination with physical exercise. If you follow a diet that normalizes the metabolism, then the need for weight loss will disappear.

__Dear friend, thanks for buying and reading my book! Please leave an honest review on the page of the book!__